Contents

INTRODUCTION

Silent reflux, also known as laryngopharyngeal reflux (LPR), is a condition characterized by the backflow of stomach contents into the throat, larynx (voice box), and nasal passages. Unlike gastroesophageal reflux disease (GERD), which is characterized by heartburn and regurgitation, silent reflux often presents with more subtle symptoms such as hoarseness, chronic cough, throat clearing, and a feeling of a lump in the throat.

The Silent Reflux Diet is a dietary approach aimed at reducing the symptoms of LPR and preventing further damage to the throat and vocal cords. This diet is based on the principle of avoiding foods and beverages that can trigger or exacerbate reflux.

One of the primary goals of the Silent Reflux Diet is to reduce the production of stomach acid. This is achieved by avoiding acidic foods and beverages, such as citrus fruits, tomatoes, vinegar, and carbonated drinks. Additionally, spicy and fried foods are often restricted as they can irritate the esophagus and trigger reflux.

Another key aspect of the Silent Reflux Diet is to limit the consumption of foods that can delay stomach emptying or relax the lower esophageal sphincter (LES), the muscle that separates the esophagus from the stomach. These include fatty and fried foods, chocolate, caffeine, alcohol, and mint.

The Silent Reflux Diet emphasizes the consumption of low-acid, easily digestible foods. These include lean protein sources such as chicken, turkey, fish, and tofu. Complex carbohydrates like whole grains, potatoes, and legumes are also recommended as they can help neutralize stomach acid. Non-citrus fruits, such as bananas, melons, and pears, are typically well-tolerated.

In addition to dietary changes, the Silent Reflux Diet may also involve lifestyle modifications. These can include eating smaller, more frequent meals, avoiding tight-fitting clothing that can put pressure on the stomach, and maintaining a healthy weight. Elevating the head of the bed and avoiding lying down for at least two to three hours after eating can also help prevent reflux episodes.

It's important to note that the Silent Reflux Diet is not a one-size-fits-all approach. Individual triggers and sensitivities can vary, and it may take some trial and error to identify the specific foods and beverages that exacerbate symptoms. Keeping a food diary and working closely with a healthcare professional or a registered dietitian can help tailor the diet to individual needs.

While the Silent Reflux Diet can be an effective management strategy for LPR, it's crucial to address the underlying causes of the condition. In some cases, medication or even surgical intervention may be necessary, particularly if dietary changes alone do not provide sufficient relief.

In conclusion, the Silent Reflux Diet is a dietary approach designed to alleviate the symptoms of laryngopharyngeal reflux and protect the throat and vocal cords from further damage. By limiting acidic, fatty, and trigger foods, and promoting the consumption of low-acid, easily digestible alternatives, the Silent Reflux Diet can help individuals manage their condition and improve their overall quality of life.

WHAT IS THE SILENT REFLUX DIET?

The silent reflux diet is an alternative treatment that can relieve symptoms of reflux with simple dietary changes. This diet is a change in lifestyle that eliminates or limits trigger foods that are known to irritate the throat or weaken the esophageal muscles.

As opposed to acid reflux or GERD, silent reflux (laryngopharyngeal reflux) may not manifest symptoms until later stages.

If you have been diagnosed with silent reflux, you may experience symptoms such as:

• sore throat

• hoarseness

• difficulty swallowing

• asthma

NUTRITION AND SILENT REFLUX

The diet plan designed for silent reflux aims to eliminate meals that exacerbate reflux symptoms and relax your esophagus. This passage, also known as the esophageal sphincter, serves as a barrier against the backward movement of food and stomach acid.

When this sphincter fails to close adequately due to relaxation, it leads to reflux symptoms.

Making dietary adjustments is crucial in preventing reflux symptoms and identifying trigger foods, which, when consumed alongside medication, can worsen your condition.

The silent reflux diet is similar to other balanced diets that are usually high in fiber, lean proteins, and vegetables. A 2004 study showed that increasing fiber and limiting salt in your diet can protect against reflux symptoms.

Some of these foods include:

• lean meats

• whole grains

• bananas

• apples

• caffeine-free beverages

• water

• leafy green vegetables

• legumes

Modifying the diet can help improve silent reflux.

One 2020 study found that people with silent reflux who eat a diet that is low in protein but high in sugary, acidic, and fatty foods experience more episodes of reflux than people who adjust their diet to increase their intake of protein.

Some foods high in protein include:

- eggs

- nuts

- seeds

- fish

Some foods low in acid include:

- fresh coconuts

- lean meat

- ginger

- oatmeal

- egg whites

To follow a diet low in sugar, a person can:

- Read the labels of food products and avoid foods containing any type of sugar or corn syrup.

- Choose brown bread or rice over white variants, as these contain simple carbohydrates.

• Opt for whole foods, such as whole grains, fish, and nuts.

To follow a diet low in fat, a person can:

• Opt for fat-free or low fat dairy products.

• Opt for wholegrain foods.

• Fill up on fruits, vegetables, or sources of lean protein.

Drinks

Medical experts recommend that people with silent reflux drink water or herbal teas.

Plant-based diet

Following a plant-based diet involves abstaining from foods containing animal products, with permissible items including vegetables, fruits, whole grains, and nuts.

A study conducted in 2017 with 184 participants revealed noteworthy findings. Ninety-nine participants adhered to a plant-based, Mediterranean-style diet comprising the aforementioned foods for six weeks, along with receiving standard treatment for silent reflux and consuming alkaline water.

The remaining 85 participants utilized both proton pump inhibitors (PPIs) and the same standard treatment for infant reflux during the same period. Upon study completion, all participants experienced a similar reduction in symptoms. The study concluded that adopting a plant-based, Mediterranean-style diet and consuming alkaline water resulted in symptom reduction comparable to conventional medications.

This approach could offer financial savings, mitigate the risk of side effects, and provide additional health benefits associated with adopting a plant-based diet.

FOODS TO AVOID

If you decide to pursue the silent reflux diet, doctors recommend eliminating high-fat foods, sweets, and acidic beverages.

Some foods to avoid include:

• whole-fat dairy products

• fried foods

• fatty cuts of meat

• caffeine

• alcohol

• sodas

• onions

• kiwi

- oranges

- limes

- lemons

- grapefruit

- pineapples

- tomatoes and tomato-based foods

It's also important to avoid chocolate, mints, and spicy foods because they're known to weaken the esophageal sphincter.

However, each trigger food can affect people differently. Pay close attention to what foods cause you more discomfort or worsen your upper endoscopy results.

Several foods may aggravate a person's silent reflux symptoms.

A person may wish to avoid the following items:

- alcohol

- chocolates

- caffeine

- peppermints

They may also wish to avoid carbonated beverages such as soda and beer, as these can weaken the lower sphincter that holds stomach acid back.

Also, acidic foods can cause stomach acid to rise into the throat.

These include:

- tomatoes

- kiwis

- pineapples

- spicy foods

Some foods can irritate the lining of the esophagus. These include fried or fatty foods, **such as:**

- fries

- chocolate

- pastries

- cheese

Also, spicy deli meats and hot spices — including mustard, curry, and hot peppers — can directly irritate the throat lining.

EATING HABITS

As well as a person changing the food they eat, they can also make adjustments to the way they eat and live to reduce silent reflux.

For example, a person with silent reflux may wish to:

• Avoid bending over within 2 hours of eating.

• Eat smaller meals throughout the day instead of three big meals.

• Avoid lying down within 3 hours of eating.

• Avoid eating or drinking anything before going to bed.

• Inserting a 4-inch wedge under the bed to elevate the head when sleeping.

RECIPE IDEAS

There are several potential ways to include generally healthy foods in small meals throughout the day.

Breakfast

For breakfast, a person may wish to consider eating oatmeal or another wholegrain cereal. Wholegrain cereals can be filling, which means that a person will need less to feel full until lunch.

People can add non-citric fruits such as coconut flakes to their oatmeal for added flavor.

Lunch

For lunch, a person may wish to consider a grilled chicken breast salad. The grilled chicken breast provides lean protein that can be filling.

Snacks

Eating snacks can help a person feel full throughout the day. A person can incorporate these to ensure that they are eating smaller meals throughout the day instead of only three larger meals.

A person could eat one hard-boiled egg or a piece of nonacidic fruit, such as melon.

Crackers and hummus may also satisfy hunger without causing additional stomach acid to form.

Dinner

A person may consume grilled fish filled with prepared vegetables, such as broccoli, for a substantial meal that wouldn't worsen silent reflux.

A person should try to include a variety of healthy foods while planning meals, such as protein sources, whole grains, vegetables, and fruits.

Dessert

For dessert, a person can choose foods such as:

• fruit ices

• nonacidic fruits

• gelatin products

OTHER AT-HOME REMEDIES

According to medical professionals, a person with silent reflux can also try:

• not smoking or using tobacco

• not wearing clothing that is too tight

• lying on the left side instead of the right

• chewing gum containing bicarbonate of soda

• maintaining a moderate weight

• taking any prescribed medication as a doctor instructs

SILENT REFLUX DIET COOKBOOK

BREAKFAST

Gluten-Free Morning Oatmeal

Makes 2 servings | 245 calories per serving

Ingredients

• 1 cup water

• 1 cup soymilk (almond or hemp milk work well, too)

• Pinch of salt

• 1 cup gluten-free rolled oats

• 2 tablespoons maple syrup

Direction

1. In a saucepan, heat up the water and soymilk with the salt.

2. Add the oats and bring to a boil, then lower the heat and cook for 10 minutes, stirring regularly.

3. Add the maple syrup before serving.

Corn Rye Savory Waffles

Makes 4–6 servings | 185 calories per serving

Ingredients

- 1 cup rye flour

- 1 cup cornmeal

- ½ teaspoon sea salt

- 1 teaspoon baking powder

- ½ teaspoon baking soda

- 2 tablespoons grapeseed oil

- 2 cups soymilk

Direction

1. In one bowl, whisk together the dry ingredients.

2. In a separate bowl, whisk together the wet ingredients.

3. Add the wet ingredients to the dry and stir gently, leaving some lumps. (Overmixing will make the waffle rubbery.)

4. Pour ¾ cup of the batter into an oiled waffle iron and cook until done.

Berry Banana Smoothie

Makes two 1-cup servings | 150 calories per serving

Ingredients

- 2 bananas

- 1 cup fresh or frozen berries

- ½ cup water

- ½ cup crushed ice

Direction

1. Add all of the ingredients to a blender and blend until smooth.

A Very Peachy Smoothie

Makes two 1-cup servings | 190 calories per serving

Ingredients

- 2 bananas

- 2 ripe peaches, peeled, halved, and pitted

- ½ cup water

- ½ cup crushed ice

Direction

1. Add all of the ingredients to a blender and blend until smooth.

SOUPS

Corn Chowder

Makes 4 servings | 195 calories per serving

Ingredients

- 2 tablespoons olive oil

- 2 teaspoons sea salt

- Kernels from 2 ears corn

- 2 medium potatoes, ¼-inch dice

- 1 large carrot, ¼-inch dice

- 1 stalk celery, finely diced

- 1 cup fresh shelled peas

- 4 cups seaweed-mushroom stock

- 1 sprig fresh rosemary

- 2 tablespoons chopped fresh parsley

- ¼ cup chopped fresh basil

- Smoked paprika,

Direction

1. In a hot soup pot, add the olive oil, sea salt, and all the vegetables. Sauté over medium heat for 10 minutes.

2. Add the stock and rosemary sprig and bring to a boil, then reduce the heat and let simmer for 3 minutes, or until the vegetables are fully cooked.

3. Add the parsley and basil and adjust the salt if needed.

4. Garnish with smoked paprika.

Borscht

Makes 4 servings | 75 calories per serving

Ingredients

- 2 pounds purple beets (3 large), peeled, ½-inch dice

- 1 tablespoon grapeseed oil

- 1 teaspoon sea salt

- 2 tablespoons chopped fresh dill

- 3 cups water

- 1-inch piece fresh horseradish, grated, or 1 teaspoon dried horseradish powder

- 2 teaspoons balsamic vinegar (optional)

Direction

1. Preheat the oven to 425°F.

2. Place the beets in a roasting pan with the oil and salt. Stir to coat well. Cover and roast for 30 minutes.

3. Combine the roasted beets, dill, water, horseradish, and balsamic vinegar in a blender and purée until smooth.

4. Chill and serve very cold in the summer, or bring to a simmer and serve hot in the winter.

Wonderful Wild Mushroom Soup

Makes 4 servings | 225 calories per serving

Ingredients

- ⅓ cup raw pine nuts

- 4 cups vegetable stock

- 3 tablespoons olive oil

- 1 stalk celery, diced

- 1 pound wild mushrooms, chopped

- 1 sprig fresh thyme

- 10 fresh sage leaves, chopped

- 2 teaspoons sea salt

- 2 tablespoons dry sherry

- Chopped fresh parsley, for garnish

Direction

1. Blend the pine nuts and stock in a blender until puréed and totally smooth. Set aside.

2. In a hot soup pot, add the olive oil.

3. Add the celery and mushrooms, thyme, sage, and sea salt, and cook until the mushrooms start to wilt.

4. Add the sherry and cook until the alcohol flavor is gone.

5. Pour in the blended pine nut and stock mixture and bring to a simmer, stirring often.

6. Season to taste and garnish with fresh parsley.

Caribbean Pumpkin Soup

Makes 4 servings | 300 calories per serving

There are two steps to this recipe, the stock and the soup; the stock can be made in advance.

Stock

- 1 small sugar pie pumpkin (also called pie pumpkin)

- 1 stalk celery, coarsely chopped

- 1 carrot, peeled and coarsely chopped

- 1 large onion, peeled and coarsely chopped

- 1 medium-size potato, peeled and coarsely chopped

- 2 whole cloves

- 1 stick cinnamon

- 1 sprig fresh thyme

- 5 allspice berries

- 2 quarts water

- 1 teaspoon sea salt

Directions for the Stock

1. Peel the pumpkin and remove the seeds and reserve; save the meat of the pumpkin for the soup.

2. Place the pumpkin peel and seeds in a stockpot, along with the celery, carrot, onion, potato, cloves, cinnamon, thyme, allspice, water, and salt.

3. Bring to a boil, then reduce the heat, cover, and let simmer for 2 hours. The liquid will reduce by half.

4. Strain the stock and reserve; discard the solid parts.

Soup

- 2 tablespoons olive oil

- Pumpkin meat reserved from making stock, diced

- 1 small parsnip, diced

- 1 carrot, diced

- 1 small potato, diced

- 1 stalk celery, diced

- 1 teaspoon sea salt

- 2 tablespoons chopped fresh parsley

Directions for the Soup

1. In a hot soup pot, add the olive oil, then add the vegetables and sea salt.

2. Over medium heat, stirring often, cook the vegetables for 10 minutes, adding a little stock if they start to stick.

3. Purée half the vegetables with the stock in a blender, leaving the remaining vegetables intact.

4. Add the puréed vegetables and stock to the solid vegetables and bring to a boil over medium heat, stirring regularly.

5. Garnish with the chopped parsley.

Miso Soup

Makes 2 servings | 50 calories per serving

Ingredients

• 2 cups seaweed-mushroom stock

• ¼ cup combination of chopped vegetables, tofu, mushrooms, and rehydrated wakame seaweed

• 4 teaspoons miso

Direction

1. Bring the stock to a simmer in a saucepan.

2. Add the vegetables, tofu, mushrooms, and seaweed and cook for 1 minute.

3. Remove from the heat.

4. Remove 2 tablespoons stock and add to a bowl with the miso. Whisk together to dissolve the miso.

5. Add the miso and stock mixture back to the rest of the soup.

6. Stir and serve immediately.

Tuscan White Bean Soup

Makes 4 servings | 400 calories per serving

Ingredients

- ¼ cup olive oil

- 1 stalk celery, diced

- 1 carrot, diced

- 1 cup fresh shelled peas

- 2 teaspoons sea salt

- 2 bay leaves

- 1 teaspoon dried oregano

- 1 teaspoon dried thyme

- ½ teaspoon dried rosemary

- ¼ cup dry white wine

- 4 cups seaweed-mushroom or vegetable stock

- 1 can white beans, rinsed and drained

- 1 cup chopped fresh basil

- ¼ cup chopped fresh parsley (preferably Italian)

Direction

1. In a large soup pot, add the olive oil.

2. Add the vegetables, salt, bay leaves, and dried herbs and cook for 10 minutes.

3. Add the white wine and cook for another 5 minutes.

4. Add the stock and beans, bring to a simmer, then season to taste.

5. Remove the bay leaves and add the basil and parsley.

Shrimp & Tofu Soup

Makes 4–6 servings | 270 calories per serving

Ingredients

- 2 tablespoons olive oil

- 4 (⅛-inch-thick) slices fresh ginger (no need to peel)

- ½ pound uncooked shrimp, peeled, deveined, and coarsely chopped (¼- to ½-inch pieces)

- ½ teaspoon rice wine

- 6 cups chicken stock

- ½ cup sliced canned bamboo shoots

- 1 (12-ounce) package soft tofu, cut into 1-inch cubes

- 2 ounces prosciutto, diced

- ¼ cup water

- ¼ cup cornstarch

- 3 egg whites, beaten

- Salt to taste

- 1 tablespoon sesame oil

- 2 tablespoons chopped fresh cilantro

Direction

1. Heat the olive oil in a pan over medium-high heat. Sauté the ginger for 2 minutes.

2. Add the shrimp and rice wine and cook until opaque. Remove from the heat, discard the ginger, and set the shrimp aside.

3. Bring the chicken stock to a boil in a saucepan over medium-high heat. Add the bamboo shoot, tofu, prosciutto, and shrimp and bring back to a boil.

4. Whisk together the water and cornstarch and slowly add the mixture to the pot while stirring constantly.

5. Slowly drizzle in the egg whites while stirring. Add salt to taste.

6. Drizzle with the sesame oil, top with the cilantro, and serve.

Asparagus Miso Chowder

Makes 4 servings | 230 calories per serving

Ingredients

• 3 medium-size red potatoes or other creamy potato, diced into ½-inch cubes

• 2 tablespoons olive oil

• 1 pound asparagus, trimmed and cut into ½-inch pieces

• ¼ cup white miso

• 4 cups vegetable or seaweed-mushroom stock

• ½ teaspoon smoked paprika for garnish (optional)

Direction

1. In a soup pot, sauté the potatoes in the olive oil over medium heat until the potatoes are soft.

2. Add the asparagus and cook for 3 more minutes.

3. Place half of the cooked vegetables in a blender and add the miso and stock.

4. Purée until very smooth.

5. Place the purée back into the pot with the solid cooked vegetables and stir to combine.

6. Serve in bowls and garnish each with a small amount of smoked paprika.

Basic Indian Bean Soup

Makes 4 servings | 210 calories per serving

Ingredients

- 6 cups water

- 2 tablespoons olive oil

- ⅔ cup dried whole mung beans

- 1 tablespoon minced fresh ginger

- ½ teaspoon ground turmeric

- 2 teaspoons ground coriander

- 1 teaspoon cumin seeds

- 1 teaspoon brown mustard seeds

- 1 ½ teaspoons salt

- ¼ teaspoon asafoetida

- 3 tablespoons chopped fresh cilantro

Direction

1. In a soup pot, bring the water to a boil.

2. Add ½ tablespoon olive oil and the mung beans, ginger, turmeric, and coriander.

3. Bring to a simmer, cover, lower the heat, and cook for 1 hour and 15 minutes.

4. In a hot frying pan or wok, add the remaining 1 ½ tablespoons olive oil.

5. Add the cumin seeds and mustard seeds and stir-fry for 30 seconds.

6. Add this to the dal soup, then add the salt, asafoetida, and cilantro.

7. Whisk the soup together to combine.

8. Cover for 1 minute and then serve hot.

Southern Black-Eyed Pea Soup

Makes 4 servings | 155 calories per serving

Ingredients

• 1 cup black-eyed peas, soaked overnight or for at least 8 hours

• 1 tablespoon olive oil

• 1 carrot, diced

• 1 stalk celery, diced

• 1 bunch collard greens, chopped

• 1 teaspoon dried thyme

• 1 teaspoon dried oregano

• 4 cups seaweed-mushroom or vegetable stock

• ½ teaspoon sea salt

• 2 tablespoons balsamic vinegar, MMGF

• ¼ cup chopped fresh parsley

Direction

1. Drain and rinse the soaked black-eyed peas.

2. In a hot soup pot, add the olive oil.

3. Add the carrot, celery, and collards and sauté for 5 minutes.

4. Add the thyme, oregano, black-eyed peas, and stock and bring to a boil.

5. Lower the heat, cover, and simmer for 25 minutes, or until the black-eyed peas are soft.

6. Stir in the salt, vinegar, and parsley.

Egg White Wrap with Dill or Basil

Makes 2 servings | 270 calories per serving

Ingredients

- 6 egg whites

- 2 tablespoons chopped fresh dill or basil

- ¼ teaspoon salt

- 1 tablespoon olive oil

- 2 flour tortillas

Direction

1. Beat the egg whites with the dill or basil and the salt.

2. Heat the oil in a small pan over medium-high heat. Add the egg mixture and scramble until cooked through.

3. Heat each tortilla in a skillet for 30 seconds to soften and to bring out the flavor.

4. Divide the egg mixture between the tortillas and roll.

Rice Porridge with Chicken

Makes 4 servings | 325 calories per serving

Ingredients

- 4 dried shiitake mushrooms

- 2 tablespoons olive oil

- 1 teaspoon minced fresh ginger

- ½ pound ground chicken

- 4 cups chicken stock

- 2 cups cooked white rice

- Salt to taste

- 2 tablespoons chopped fresh cilantro

- 1 teaspoon sesame oil

Direction

1. In warm water soak the mushrooms until soft.

2. Rinse the mushrooms and pat dry.

3. Remove the stems and thinly slice the caps.

4. Heat the olive oil in a pan over medium-high heat. Add the ginger and sauté for 1 minute. Add the mushrooms and ground chicken and sauté until the chicken is browned. Remove from the heat and set aside.

5. Bring the chicken stock to a boil in a saucepan over medium-high heat.

6. Add the cooked white rice and return to a boil, then reduce the heat to low and cook until soft, about 15 minutes.

7. Add the chicken and mushroom mixture and cook another 5 minutes, then add salt to taste.

8. Pour into bowls, top with the cilantro, drizzle with the sesame oil, and serve.

Buckwheat Waffles

Makes 4 servings | 165 calories per serving

Ingredients

- ½ cup buckwheat flour

- ½ cup white flour

- 1 tablespoon palm sugar

- ¼ teaspoon baking soda

- ½ teaspoon baking powder

- 1 teaspoon vanilla extract

- 1 tablespoon grapeseed oil

- 1 cup soymilk (see note)

Direction

1. In one bowl, whisk together the dry ingredients.

2. In another bowl, whisk together the wet ingredients.

3. Add the wet ingredients to the dry and stir gently, leaving some lumps. (Overmixing will make the waffle rubbery.)

4. Pour ¾ cup of the batter into an oiled waffle iron and cook until done.

Gluten-Free Pumpkin Muffins

Makes 12 muffins | 130 calories per muffin

Ingredients

- ⅓ cup quinoa flour

- ½ cup quinoa flakes

- 1 teaspoon baking soda

- 2 teaspoons baking powder

- 1 teaspoon ground cinnamon

- ½ teaspoon ground ginger

- ¼ teaspoon ground cloves

- 2–3 tablespoons honey (optional)

- 2 eggs

- 2 ripe bananas, mashed

- 1 cup pumpkin purée (from can)

Direction

1. Preheat the oven to 400°F.

2. In one bowl, whisk together the quinoa flour, quinoa flakes, baking soda, baking powder, cinnamon, ginger, cloves, and salt.

3. In another bowl, whisk together the honey, eggs, bananas, and pumpkin.

4. Add the banana mixture to the flour mixture and stir gently.

5. Prepare a 12-muffin tin by spraying it with nonstick cooking spray (or coating it with grapeseed oil).

6. Divide the mixture between the muffin cups and bake for 25 minutes.

Supa-Dupa Vegan Frittata

Ingredients

• 1 (16-ounce) package medium-firm tofu

• ½ cup soymilk

• 1¼ teaspoons sea salt

• 1 tablespoon cornstarchMMGF

• ½ teaspoon ground turmeric

• 1 teaspoon olive oil, plus as needed

• 2 cups mixed chopped vegetables (mushrooms, spinach, red pepper, or anything you like that is in season)

• 2 tablespoons chopped fresh basil

• 1 teaspoon fresh thyme, or ½ teaspoon dried thyme

Direction

1. Press the tofu by removing it from the package and placing it on a towel. Place another towel on the tofu and then a cutting board on top of this towel. Place a heavy can or another heavy item from your kitchen on the board. Let the tofu press for 10 minutes. Pressing the tofu will remove the water and allow it to absorb other flavors.

2. Place the tofu, soymilk, 1 teaspoon sea salt, cornstarch, and turmeric in a blender or food processor and purée until very smooth. Set aside.

3. Heat up a frying pan over medium heat and add the olive oil.

4. Add the vegetables and the remaining ¼ teaspoon sea salt.

5. Cook over medium heat, stirring regularly, until the vegetables are starting to wilt. Remove the cooked vegetables from the pan and set aside.

6. In the same frying pan, coat the surface with a little more olive oil.

7. Pour ¾ cup of the tofu-soymilk mixture into the pan, spreading evenly.

8. Cover and cook for 7 minutes, or until the surface is dry.

9. Add the cooked vegetables to the top of one side of the cooked tofu mixture.

10. Using a spatula, gently remove the frittata from the surface of the pan and fold one half over the side with the vegetables.

11. Sprinkle with the herbs and serve hot.

Gluten-Free Caramel Apple Muffins

Makes 12 muffins | 125 calories per muffin

Ingredients

- ⅓ cup quinoa flour

- ½ cup quinoa flakes

- 1 teaspoon baking soda

- 2 teaspoons baking powder

- 1 teaspoon ground cinnamon

- ½ teaspoon ground nutmeg

- ½ teaspoon salt

- ½ cup caramel candy bits

- 1 teaspoon milk

- 1 cup diced red apple

- 2 tablespoons honey

- 2 eggs

- 2 very ripe bananas, mashed

Direction

1. Preheat the oven to 400°F.

2. In one bowl, whisk together the quinoa flour, quinoa flakes, baking soda, baking powder, cinnamon, nutmeg, and salt.

3. Heat a nonstick saucepan over medium heat and spray with nonstick cooking spray (or coat with grapeseed oil), then turn the heat to low. Add the caramel and milk and stir until

the caramel is melted and smooth. Add the apples and stir for 1 minute. Remove from the heat and keep warm. (If the mixture hardens before use, you can microwave it in a microwave-safe bowl on high for 30 seconds.)

4. In another bowl, whisk together the honey, eggs, bananas, and caramel apple mixture.

5. Add the caramel mixture to the flour mixture and stir gently.

6. Prepare a 12-muffin tin by spraying it with nonstick cooking spray (or coating it with grapeseed oil).

7. Divide the mixture between the muffin cups and bake for 20–25 minutes.

Chicken-Stuffed Cucumber Soup
Makes 8 servings | 230 calories per serving

Ingredients

Marinade

- 1 egg white

- 1 tablespoon minced fresh ginger

- 2 tablespoons water

- 1 teaspoon salt

- 1 teaspoon tamari (gluten-free soy sauce)

- ¼ teaspoon honey

- 1 tablespoon cornstarch

- Dash of toasted sesame oil

Soup

- 1 pound ground chicken

- 2 tablespoons cornstarch

- 2 medium cucumbers, peeled, seeded to make a hollow area, and sliced cross wise into 2-inch pieces

- 8 cups chicken stock

- 2 (¼-inch-thick) slices peeled fresh ginger, diced

- 1 teaspoon salt

- 8 shiitake or portobello mushrooms, trimmed and sliced

- 10 sprigs fresh cilantro, chopped, for garnish

- 4 teaspoons sesame oil

Direction

1. Combine all of the marinade ingredients in a bowl.

2. Add the ground chicken, mix well, and let marinate for 5 minutes.

3.   Lightly dust the cornstarch inside the cucumber pieces.

4. Stuff each hollowed-out area of cucumber with chicken mixture.

5. Bring the chicken stock to a boil in a soup pot over medium-high heat, then add the sliced ginger and salt.

6. Add the stuffed cucumber pieces, bring back to a boil, then lower the heat to medium-low and gently boil for 10–15 minutes, or until the chicken is cooked through.

7. Add the mushrooms and simmer for 1 minute.

8. Serve hot with the chopped cilantro and a drizzle of sesame oil.

SALADS

Spanish Bean Salad

Makes 6 servings | 290 calories per serving

Ingredients

- ¼ pound green beans, trimmed and cut into ½-inch pieces

- 1 (16-ounce) can garbanzo beans

- 1 (16-ounce) can kidney beans

- 1 (16-ounce) can black-eyed peas

- 1 large carrot, grated

- 1 teaspoon dried rosemary

- 2 teaspoons dried oregano

- 1 teaspoon dried thyme

- 3 tablespoons olive oil

- 3 tablespoons sherry vinegar

- 2 teaspoons sea salt

- 1 teaspoon mustard powder

- 1 tablespoon lemon zest

- ¼ cup chopped fresh parsley

Direction

1. Blanch the green beans by dropping them in boiling water for 5 seconds. Rinse under cold water and drain.

2. Rinse the 3 cans of beans well and drain.

3. Place all of the ingredients in a large bowl and mix well.

4. Let marinate for 2 hours before serving.

Cucumber Wakame Salad

Makes 4 servings | 20 calories per serving

Ingredients

- 1 cucumber, cut into ⅛-inch-thick slices

- ½ teaspoon salt

- 2 tablespoons dried wakame

- 1 cup cold water

- 1 carrot, grated

- 2 teaspoons rice vinegar

- 1 teaspoon mirin

- 1 teaspoon tamari (gluten-free soy sauce)

Direction

1. Place the cucumber slices in a colander set over a bowl, sprinkle with the salt, and massage it into the slices. Let the cucumber sit in the colander for 30 minutes, then rinse and drain.

2. Meanwhile, rehydrate the wakame by placing it in the cold water for 15 minutes. Drain and squeeze excess water out of the wakame.

3. Place the cucumber and wakame with the remaining ingredients in a bowl and gently mix. Serve immediately.

Roasted Portobello Mushroom Salad
Makes 4 servings | 115 calories per serving

Ingredients

- 2 portobello mushrooms

- 1 tablespoon olive oil

- ¼ teaspoon sea salt

- 1 large bunch arugula, chopped

- ½ head radicchio, shredded

Dressing

- 2 tablespoons olive oil

- 2 tablespoons balsamic vinegar

- ¼ teaspoon dried thyme

- ¼ teaspoon dried rosemary

- ¼ teaspoon dried oregano

- ¼ teaspoon dried sage

- ¼ cup chopped fresh parsley

- 1 teaspoon sea salt

Direction

1. Preheat the oven to 400°F.

2. Trim the stems off the mushrooms, then lightly rinse the mushrooms and pat dry. Scoop out the gills.

3. Brush the mushrooms on all sides with the olive oil and rub a little salt into them.

4. Place on a baking sheet and roast for 10 minutes. Then turn them over and roast another 10 minutes.

5. Slice the mushrooms and arrange on top of a bed of arugula and radicchio.

6. In a separate bowl, whisk together the dressing ingredients and pour the dressing over the mushrooms and greens.

Roasted Corn with Cilantro & Lime Zest

Makes 4 servings | 115 calories per serving

Ingredients

- Kernels from 4 ears corn

- 1 teaspoon sea salt

- 1 tablespoon grapeseed oil

- ¼ cup chopped fresh cilantro

- 2 tablespoons chopped fresh sage

- 2 tablespoons lime zest

- 2 tablespoons balsamic vinegar

Direction

1. Preheat the oven to 425°F.

2. Combine the corn with the salt and oil and place in a roasting pan.

3. Roast, covered, for 30 minutes, or until the corn is slightly caramelized.

4. Transfer the corn to a bowl and add the rest of the ingredients. Stir to combine and serve warm or at room temperature.

Dandelions with Garlic-Oil Dressing

Makes 4 servings | 80 calories per serving

Ingredients

- 1 large bunch dandelions, chopped

- 2 tablespoons garlic-infused olive oil

- 1 teaspoon rice vinegar

- ½ teaspoon sea salt

Direction

1. Blanch the dandelions by dropping them in boiling water for a few seconds. Rinse with cold water, drain, and squeeze out excess water.

2. Place the dandelions in a bowl and add the rest of the ingredients. Toss to combine and let sit for an hour before serving.

Spinach with Sesame Dressing

Makes 4 servings | 85 calories per serving

Ingredients

- 1 pound fresh spinach leaves

- ¼ cup toasted sesame seeds

- 1 tablespoon seaweed-mushroom stock

- 1½ tablespoons tamari (gluten-free soy sauce)

- 1 teaspoon sake

- 1 tablespoon mirin

Direction

1. Blanch the spinach by dropping it in boiling water for a few seconds. Then immediately drain it and rinse the spinach under cold water. Squeeze all water out of the spinach and set aside.

2. In a mortar and pestle or a food processor, grind the sesame seeds down.

3. Combine the stock, tamari, sake, mirin, and ground sesame seeds in a bowl.

4. Coat the spinach with the sesame seed dressing.

Wilted Kale Salad

Makes 4 servings | 115 calories per serving

Ingredients

- 1 bunch kale, stalks removed, leaves chopped very small

- 1 tablespoon balsamic vinegar

- ½ teaspoon sea salt

- 1 carrot, grated

- 1 tablespoon lemon zest

- 1 tablespoon toasted pumpkin seeds

- 1 teaspoon mirin

- 1 tablespoon olive oil

Direction

1. Place the kale in a bowl and massage the balsamic vinegar and salt into the kale. Let sit for 30 minutes.

2. Add the rest of the ingredients and mix well to coat the kale leaves.

French Lentil Salad

Makes 4 servings | 165 calories per serving

Ingredients

- 1 cup green lentils, soaked overnight or for at least 8 hours

- 1 quart boiling water

- 1 tablespoon olive oil

- 1 carrot, diced

- 1 stalk celery, diced

- 1 cup fresh shelled peas

- ½ teaspoon dried thyme

- ½ teaspoon dried oregano

- ½ teaspoon dried marjoram

- ½ teaspoon dried rosemary

- 1 teaspoon sea salt

- 2 tablespoons lemon zest

- ¼ cup chopped fresh parsley or basil

- 2 tablespoons balsamic vinegar

Direction

1. Drain and rinse the soaked lentils.

2. Cook the lentils in the boiling water for 10 minutes, or until the lentils are soft. Do not overcook!

3. Drain the lentils well and set aside in a bowl.

4. In a hot frying pan, add the olive oil, vegetables, dried herbs, and salt. Sauté for 5 minutes, or until the vegetables are cooked.

5. Add the cooked vegetables to the cooked lentils, then add the lemon zest, parsley, and balsamic vinegar and toss well to combine.

Hijiki Seaweed Salad

Makes 4 servings | 85 calories per serving

Ingredients

- ½ ounce dried hijiki

- 1 quart water

- 1 carrot, julienned

- 2 tablespoons sake

- 2 tablespoons mirin

- 2 tablespoons tamari (gluten-free soy sauce)

- 1 cup seaweed-mushroom stock

- ½ cup fresh or frozen shelled edamame

- 1 tablespoon toasted sesame seeds (optional)

Direction

1. Reconstitute the hijiki by soaking it in the water for 30 minutes. Drain and rinse.

2. Place the hijiki with the carrot, sake, mirin, tamari, and stock in a pot and bring to a simmer.

3. Cover, lower the heat, and cook for 30 minutes.

4. Add the edamame and cook another 10 minutes, adding more stock if needed.

5. Garnish with the toasted sesame seeds.

Makes 4 servings | 290 calories per serving

Ingredients

- 1 (16-ounce) can garbanzo beans, drained and rinsed

- 2 tablespoons high-quality olive oil or garlic-infused olive oil

- 2 tablespoons lemon zest

- 3 tablespoons tahini

- 1 teaspoon ground cumin

- ½ teaspoon ground coriander

- 1 teaspoon sea salt

- 1 teaspoon sumac

- 2 tablespoons chopped fresh dill, or 1 teaspoon dried dill

- 1 cucumber, thinly sliced

- 1 carrot, grated

- ½ cup alfalfa or radish sprouts

Direction

1. In a food processor, add the beans, olive oil, lemon zest, tahini, cumin, coriander, salt, sumac, and dill and purée until very smooth.

2. Transfer the hummus to a bowl. Place the sliced cucumbers around the sides, pile the grated carrots in the middle, and top with the sprouts.

SIDES

Pickled Bean Sprouts

Makes 4 servings | 45 calories per serving

Ingredients

- 3 cups water

- ⅛ teaspoon baking soda

- 1 pound mung bean or soybean sprouts

- 2 tablespoons tamari (gluten-free soy sauce)

- 1 tablespoon mirin

- 1 tablespoon rice vinegar

Direction

1. Bring the water and baking soda to a boil in a pot over medium-high heat.

2. Blanch the sprouts by dropping them in the boiling water and then immediately removing them.

3. Immediately rinse under cold water to stop the cooking process. Drain and transfer the sprouts to a bowl.

4. Add the tamari, mirin, and rice vinegar to the blanched sprouts and let marinate for 2 hours before serving.

Taiwanese Dill with Ginger

Makes 4 servings | 100 calories per serving

Ingredients

- 3 tablespoons olive oil

- 2 (¼-inch-thick) slices fresh ginger (no need to peel)

- 1 bunch dill, chopped (about 3–4 cups)

- 1 tablespoon rice wine

- ¼ cup water or seaweed-mushroom or

- vegetable stock

- Salt to taste

Direction

1. Heat the oil in a pan over medium-high heat, then add the ginger and sauté until fragrant, about 1 minute.

2. Add the dill, rice wine, water, and salt to taste and cook for 2–3 minutes. Serve hot.

Roasted Butternut Squash Purée

Makes 4 servings | 90 calories per serving

Ingredients

• 1 butternut squash, peeled, seeded, and diced

• 1 tablespoon grapeseed oil

• 1 teaspoon sea salt

Direction

1. Preheat the oven to 425°F.

2. Combine the squash, grapeseed oil, and salt in a roasting pan and mix until the squash is well coated.

3. Cover with foil and roast for 30 minutes.

4. Mash squash with a fork or a potato masher, or purée in a food processor.

Roasted Asparagus with Black Olives

Makes 4 servings | 155 calories per serving

Ingredients

• 1 pound asparagus, 2 inches trimmed off bottoms

• ¼ cup pitted and chopped black olives

• 2 tablespoons chopped fresh parsley

• 2 tablespoons white wine

• 1 tablespoon olive oil

Direction

1. Preheat the oven to 425°F.

2. Combine all of the ingredients in a bowl and mix well.

3. Place on a baking sheet in a single layer and roast, uncovered, for 15 minutes, or until asparagus is tender.

Polenta with Pistachios & Fennel
Makes 4 servings | 325 calories per serving

Ingredients

• 2 tablespoons olive oil

• ⅓ cup minced fennel bulb, ⅛-inch pieces

• 1½ teaspoons sea salt

• 1 cup polenta

• ½ cup raw pistachios

• 2 cups soymilk

- 2 cups seaweed-mushroom stock

- 2 tablespoons chopped fresh parsley

- 1 tablespoon chopped fresh basil

Direction

1. In a saucepan, add the olive oil, fennel, and sea salt and sauté for 4 minutes over medium heat.

2. Add the polenta, pistachios, soymilk, and stock and bring to a simmer over high heat.

3. Lower the heat and continue cooking for 30 minutes, stirring regularly. The polenta will thicken, so you must stir to keep it from sticking.

4. Add the parsley and basil.

5. Remove from the heat and pour the polenta into an oiled baking dish.

6. Let cool and set for 2 hours.

7. Cut pieces of polenta and eat as is or grill before serving.

Korean Cold Noodles with Soy-Sesame Milk (Kong gook soo)

Makes 4 servings | 315 calories per serving

Ingredients

- 1 cup dried soybeans

- ¼ cup raw sesame seeds

- 1 pound Korean or Japanese soba noodles

- Several ice cubes

- Salt to taste

- Daikon sprouts (kaiware), for garnish

- 1 cucumber, shredded

Direction

1. Soak the soybeans and sesame seeds in 2 quarts water overnight or for 8 hours.

2. Drain and rinse the soybeans and sesame seeds and place in a blender with 1 quart cold water. Purée until smooth. Chill until ice cold.

3. Cook the soba noodles according to the package directions. Drain and rinse under cold water until cool, then drain again.

4. Divide the soba among 4 bowls, then pour the cold soy-sesame mixture over each bowl. Add ice to each bowl.

5. Salt to taste.

6. Garnish with daikon sprouts and cucumber.

Oat Pilaf

Makes 4 servings | 200 calories per serving

Ingredients

- 1 tablespoon olive oil

- 1 stalk celery, diced

- 3 cremini, button, or shiitake mushrooms, chopped

- ⅓ cup fresh shelled peas

- 1 carrot, diced

- 1 teaspoon sea salt

- 1 cup whole dried oats

- 3 cups water or seaweed-mushroom or

- vegetable stock

- ¼ cup chopped fresh parsley

Direction

1. In a saucepan, heat up the olive oil, then add the celery, mushrooms, peas, carrots, and salt and cook for 5 minutes.

2. Add the oats and water and bring to a boil.

3. Lower the heat, cover tightly, and cook for 50 minutes. Garnish with the parsley.

Roasted Eggplant

Makes 4 servings | 65 calories per serving

Ingredients

- 1 small eggplant

- 1 teaspoon sea salt

- 1 tablespoon olive oil

Direction

1. Cut the eggplant into ½-inch-thick slices.

2. Sprinkle the salt on the eggplant slices and massage it in gently.

3. Put the eggplant in a colander set over a bowl to drain for 1 hour.

4. Preheat the oven to 425°F.

5. Brush the eggplant slices with the olive oil.

6. Roast in a single layer on a baking sheet for 15 minutes. Then turn over and roast another 10 minutes, or until the eggplant is slightly charred.

Anadama Bread

Makes 2 loaves | 95 calories per serving

Ingredients

• 1 teaspoon dry yeast

• 2 tablespoons blackstrap molasses

• 1 cup warm water (100°F)

• 1 cup soymilk

• 2 teaspoons sea salt

• 2 cups cornmeal

• 2 cups white flour

• Olive oil, for brushing

Direction

1. Add the yeast and blackstrap molasses to the warm water in a bowl and whisk.

2. Let sit for 5 minutes, until foamy.

3. Add the soymilk and sea salt and whisk together.

4. Slowly start to incorporate first the cornmeal and then the flour into the yeast mixture. At first with a spoon, and then

laying the dough on a flat surface and using your hands, knead the dough for 10 minutes, until smooth and shiny. Add more flour if it gets too sticky.

5. Brush the dough with olive oil, place in a bowl, and cover with a towel. Let sit about 1 hour, or until the dough has doubled in size.

6. Cut the dough in half, shape into loaves, and place on an oiled baking sheet or into oiled loaf pans. Cover and let rise another hour, or until doubled in size.

7. Preheat the oven to 500°F.

8. Bake loaves for 25 minutes, or until golden brown.

Salmon Fried Rice

Makes 4 servings | 375 calories per serving

Ingredients

- ¼ cup olive oil

- 8 ounces smoked salmon

- ¼ cup fresh shelled peas

- ¼ cup diced carrots, ¼-inch pieces

- 3 egg whites

- 1 egg yolk

- 3 cups cooked rice

- Salt to taste

Direction

1. Heat the oil in a pan over medium-high, then add the smoked salmon and sauté until cooked through, breaking it into bite-size pieces with a spatula while stir-frying.

2. Add the peas and carrots and cook until the carrots start to soften.

3. Whisk the egg whites and egg yolk together, then add to the pan. Scramble until cooked through.

4. Add the rice and mix well. Cook until the rice is heated through.

5. Season with salt to taste.

Fennel Roasted Beets

Makes 4 servings | 60 calories per serving

Ingredients

- 1 large purple beet, peeled and diced

- 1 small bulb fresh fennel, diced

- 1 tablespoon grapeseed oil

- 1 teaspoon sea salt

• 1 tablespoon balsamic vinegar

Direction

1. Preheat the oven to 425°F.

2. Place the diced beets and diced fennel in a roasting pan with the oil and salt. Stir to coat well. Cover and roast for 30 minutes, or until slightly browned and caramelized on the edges.

3. Toss with the balsamic vinegar and serve.

Rustic Whole-Wheat Bread
Makes 2 loaves | 100 calories per slice

Ingredients

• 1 teaspoon dry yeast

• 1 tablespoon agave

• 2 cups warm water (100°F)

• 2 teaspoons sea salt

• 2 cups white flour

• 2 cups whole-wheat flour

• 1 tablespoon olive oil

Direction

1. Add the yeast and agave to the warm water in a bowl and whisk.

2. Let sit 5 minutes, until foamy.

3. Add the sea salt and whisk.

4. Slowly start to incorporate the flours into the yeast mixture. At first with a spoon, and then laying the dough on a flat surface and using your hands, knead the dough for 10 minutes, until smooth and shiny. Add more flour if it gets too sticky.

5. Brush the dough with the olive oil, place in a bowl, and cover with a towel. Let sit about 1 hour, or until the dough has doubled in size.

6. Cut the dough in half, shape into loaves, and place on an oiled baking sheet or into oiled loaf pans. Cover and let rise another hour, or until doubled in size.

7. Preheat the oven to 500°F.

8. Bake the loaves for 25 minutes, or until golden brown.

Stir-Fried Brussels Sprouts

Makes 4 servings | 60 calories per serving

Ingredients

- About 20 Brussels sprouts

- 1 teaspoon sesame oil

- 1 tablespoon minced fresh ginger

- 1 tablespoon tamari (gluten-free soy sauce)

- 1 tablespoon mirin

- 1 tablespoon sake

- 1 teaspoon toasted sesame oil

- Cooked brown rice, for serving

Direction

1. Trim the bottom ends off the sprouts and then thinly slice.

2. In a hot wok or frying pan, add the sesame oil and ginger and stir-fry for 30 seconds.

3. Add the sprouts and stir-fry for 5 minutes.

4. Add the tamari, mirin, and sake and stir-fry for 1 minute.

5. Remove from the heat, add the toasted sesame oil, and stir well. Serve with brown rice.

Rice with Cumin & Turmeric

Makes 4 servings | 200 calories per serving

Ingredients

- 1 cup uncooked rice

- 2 cups vegetable stock

- 1 tablespoon olive oil

- 1 teaspoon sea salt

- ½ teaspoon ground cumin

- ½ teaspoon ground turmeric

Direction

1. Add all of the ingredients to a rice cooker and cook according to the manufacturer's instructions.

2. Fluff the rice with a fork and serve immediately.

Emperor's Jade Fried Rice
Makes 4 servings | 425 calories per serving

Ingredients

- 4 tablespoons olive oil

- 2 cups chopped spinach

- 2 cups chopped mustard greens

- 3 egg whites

- 1 egg yolk

- 4 cups cooked rice

- ¼ cup diced smoked tofu

- ¼-inch pieces

- Salt to taste

Direction

1. Heat 2 tablespoons of the oil in a pan over medium-high heat, then add the spinach and mustard greens and sauté until wilted. Remove from the heat and drain the excess water from the pan.

2. Remove the greens from the pan and set aside.

3. Heat the remaining 2 tablespoons oil in the same pan over medium-high heat. Whisk the egg whites and egg yolk together, then add to the pan. Scramble the eggs until cooked through.

4. Add the rice, spinach and mustard greens mixture, and smoked tofu and mix well. Cook until heated through.

5. Season with salt to taste.

Cold Somen Noodles with Dipping Sauce
Makes 4 servings | 460 calories per serving

Ingredients

Dipping sauce

- 1⅔ cups seaweed-mushroom stock

- ½ cup sake

- ¼ cup tamari (gluten-free soy sauce)

- ½ teaspoon salt

- ½ teaspoon palm sugar

- 1 pound somen noodles or angel hair pasta

- Several ice cubes

- 1 sheet nori, cut into thin shreds

- 2 teaspoons prepared wasabi

Direction

1. Place all of the sauce ingredients in a saucepan. Bring to a boil, lower the heat, and simmer for 3 minutes. Chill completely.

2. Cook the noodles according to the package directions. Drain under cold water until cool, then drain again.

3. To serve, place a couple cubes of ice into individual serving bowls. Place noodles over ice. Each person gets another bowl for the sauce.

4. Garnish the noodles with nori and wasabi.

5. To eat, take the noodles, dip in the sauce, and slurp away!

Sweet Potatoes, Cabbage & Kale

Makes 4 servings | 200 calories per serving

Ingredients

• 1 large sweet potato, peeled and chopped into 1-inch cubes

• 1 bunch kale, stalks removed, leaves chopped

• 2 tablespoons olive oil

• 3 tablespoons grated fresh ginger

• ½ head purple cabbage, chopped

• 2 tablespoons tamari (gluten-free soy sauce)

• 1 tablespoon palm sugar

• ¼ cup chopped fresh cilantro, for garnish

Direction

1. Steam the sweet potatoes and kale for 10 minutes, or until cooked.

2. In a hot frying pan, add the olive oil.

3. Add the ginger and sauté for 2 minutes.

4. Add the purple cabbage and sauté for 10 minutes.

5. Add the steamed sweet potatoes and kale, tamari, and palm sugar. Cook until heated through.

6. Garnish with the cilantro.

Yummy Roasted Mashed Root Vegetables
Makes 4 servings | 130 calories per serving

Ingredients

• 2 small potatoes, peeled and cut into 1-inch cubes

• 1 large parsnip, peeled and cut into 1-inch cubes

• 1 medium-size sweet potato (preferably satsuma imo), peeled and cut into 1-inch cubes

• 1 small celery root, peeled and cut into 1-inch cubes

• 1 tablespoon grapeseed oil

• 1 teaspoon sea salt

• ¼ cup chopped fresh parsley, for garnish

Direction

1. Preheat the oven to 425°F.

2. Toss the vegetables with the oil and salt and place in a roasting pan. Cover with foil and roast for 40 minutes, or until slightly caramelized.

3. Mash the roasted vegetables with a fork or a potato masher.

4. Garnish with the chopped parsley.

Stir-Fried Green Beans with Ginger

Makes 4 servings | 50 calories per serving

Ingredients

- 1 quart water

- ⅛ teaspoon baking soda

- 1 pound Chinese long beans or string

- beans (remove the strings if using string beans)

- 1 tablespoon shaoshing wine

- 1 teaspoon palm sugar

- 1 tablespoon sesame oil

- 1 teaspoon fermented black beans

- 3 tablespoons minced fresh ginger

Direction

1. Bring the water and baking soda to a rapid boil in a pot over high heat.

2. Drop the green beans in the boiling water for 5 seconds to blanch them. Immediately drain and rinse under cold water to stop the cooking process.

3. In a bowl, combine the shaoshing with the tamari and palm sugar and set aside.

4. In a hot wok or frying pan over medium-high heat, add the sesame oil, fermented black beans, and ginger and stir-fry for 2 minutes.

5. Add the blanched beans and stir-fry another 2 minutes.

6. Add the shaoshing mixture and cook for 10 seconds, stirring to coat.

ENTRÉES

Steamed Mussels & Shrimp Pot
Makes 3–4 servings | 450 calories per serving

Ingredients

- 3–4 tablespoons olive oil

- ½ teaspoon sea salt

- 2 shallots, diced

- 1 bulb fennel (not the green parts), coarsely chopped

- 1–2 large tomatoes, diced

- 1–2 cups chicken stock; enough to cover the bottom of your pot, ½ to 1 inch up the side)

- 4 pounds fresh mussels, scrubbed and debearded

- 1–1½ pounds fresh uncooked shrimp, shell on

- ¼ cup chopped fresh cilantro leaves, for garnish

Direction

1. Place your biggest stockpot with a lid (one that will hold all of the ingredients) over medium-high heat and add the olive oil. Then add the salt, shallots, and fennel. Sauté until soft.

2. Add the tomato and continue to cook.

3. Add the chicken stock and bring to a boil over high heat.

4. When the stock is boiling, add the mussels and shrimp and cover.

5. Every 2–3 minutes, with a large serving utensil, move the mussels and shrimp about so that the bottom ones come to the top.

6. When all of the mussels have opened (discard any that haven't), after about 10–12 minutes of steaming, garnish with cilantro and serve in big bowls.

Four-Star Marinated Smoked Tempeh

Makes 4 servings | 275 calories per serving

Ingredients

• 2 tablespoons tamari (gluten-free soy sauce)

• 1 tablespoon sesame oil

• 1 tablespoon mirin

• 1 tablespoon maple syrup

• 2 tablespoons seaweed-mushroom stock

• 1 pound tempeh (usually this will be two ½-pound packages)

• Apple wood or cherry wood, for smoking

Direction

1. Mix together all of the ingredients (except the tempeh and apple wood) in a bowl. Add the tempeh and let marinate for 1 hour.

2. Smoke over apple wood or cherry wood for about 15 minutes, or until browned and aromatic.

Makes 8–10 servings | 190 calories per serving

Ingredients

• ¼ cup olive oil

• 1–2 pork tenderloins

• 1–2 teaspoons sea salt

• Savory, ground

• Cardamom, ground

• Cumin, ground

Direction

1. Put the oil on the bottom of a large dish and add the pork tenderloins.

2. With a fork, turn the pork so that it gets lightly coated with the oil; add the salt while turning.

3. Next, sprinkle the three spices liberally on the pork, on at least two sides.

4. Cover tightly with plastic wrap and refrigerate. This meat can stay in the refrigerator for up to 2 days.

5. Preheat the grill on high and when hot, sear the tenderloins for 3–5 minutes on each side.

6. Remove the pork from the grill, cover with foil, and let rest about 5 minutes.

7. Turn ,down the heat to medium. (If your grill has a temperature gauge, you sear at about 700°F and then cook over medium at 300–400°F.)

8. When the grill is ready, put the pork back on the grill for 20–30 minutes, turning once or twice.

9. When done, place on a cutting board for a few minutes before cutting into ½-inch slices.

Pumpkin Gnocchi with Pistachio Sauce
Makes 4 servings | 380 calories per serving

Ingredients

Gnocchi

- 1 cup roasted pumpkin purée

- 1 teaspoon sea salt

- ¼ teaspoon ground nutmeg

- 1 cup semolina flour

Sauce

- 1 cup raw pistachios

- 1 teaspoon sea salt

- 2 cups soymilk

- 20 fresh sage leaves (preferably with stems attached)

- ½ teaspoon freshly grated nutmeg

Directions for the gnocchi

1. Combine the pumpkin with the salt and nutmeg and mix well. Slowly incorporate the flour until you have a dough. The less flour you add, the lighter the gnocchi will be.

2. Let the dough rest, covered or wrapped, for a half hour.

3. Divide the dough into 4 equal-size portions.

4. Roll out each portion into 1-inch-diameter logs of dough, flouring lightly as needed.

5. Cut the logs into ¾-inch-long pieces to create the gnocchi.

6. Drop the gnocchi in boiling water. When they float, they are finished. Remove from the water, drain, and sauce immediately. Do NOT make in advance; make them as you are ready to serve them.

Directions for the sauce

1. In a cast-iron skillet over medium-low heat, toast the pistachios, stirring constantly until they smell aromatic.

Remove from the heat and place in a blender with the salt and soymilk. Blend until smooth.

2. Transfer the pistachio purée into a saucepan and place over low heat.

3. Add the sage leaves and, stirring regularly, bring to a simmer. Cook, stirring, until the sauce thickens slightly.

4. Add the nutmeg, remove the sage leaves, and serve the sauce with the gnocchi.

Turkey & Mushrooms with Rice

Makes 6 servings | 445 calories per serving

Ingredients

- 6 dried shiitake mushrooms

- 3 tablespoons olive oil

- 1 tablespoon minced fresh ginger

- 1 pound ground turkey

- ½ cup rice wine

- ½ cup tamari (gluten-free soy sauce)

- 2 cups water

- 1 teaspoon sugar

- ½ teaspoon Chinese spice blend

- 1 star anise

- Cooked rice, for serving

- Chopped fresh cilantro, for garnish

- Julienned carrots, for garnish

- Bean sprouts, for garnish

Direction

1. In warm water, soak the mushrooms until soft. Rinse the mushrooms and pat dry. Remove the stems and thinly slice the caps.

2. Heat the oil in a pan over medium-high heat. Add the ginger and sauté for 1 minute. Add the mushrooms and turkey and sauté until the turkey is browned.

3. Add the wine, tamari, water, sugar, Chinese spice blend, and star anise. Bring to a boil, then lower the heat to simmer for 45 minutes.

4. Remove the star anise and discard. Serve over rice and garnish with cilantro, carrots, and bean sprouts.

One-Pot Ginger Chicken Rice
Makes 4 servings | 675 calories per serving

Ingredients

- Marinated chicken

- ⅛ teaspoon salt

- 2 tablespoons tamari (gluten-free soy sauce)

- 2 tablespoons olive oil

- 2 tablespoons rice wine

- 4 chicken breasts

- 6 dried shiitake or portobello mushrooms

- 3 tablespoons olive oil

- 12 (⅛-inch-thick) slices peeled fresh ginger

- 2 cups uncooked jasmine or other long grain rice 1½ cups chicken stock

- ¼ cup rice wine (preferably shaoshing

- Sea salt to taste

- 1–2 tablespoons tamari (gluten-free soy sauce)

- Few dashes of sesame oil

- Chopped fresh cilantro, for garnish

Direction

1. For the marinated chicken, mix the salt, tamari, olive oil, and rice wine in a large bowl. Add the chicken breasts and

marinate the chicken for 30 minutes in the refrigerator. Drain and set aside the chicken (discard the marinade).

2. In warm water, soak the mushrooms until soft. Rinse the mushrooms and pat dry. Remove the stems and thinly slice the caps.

3. Heat the oil in a pan over medium-high heat and sauté the ginger until fragrant for 1 minute.

4. Add the rice and mix well to coat with oil.

5. Add the chicken stock, rice wine, and salt to taste and mix well.

6. Transfer to a rice cooker and place the chicken breasts and mushrooms on top. Cook the rice according to the manufacturer's instructions. (Alternatively, if you don't have a rice cooker, cook in a pot on the stovetop for at least 20–25 minutes.)

7. Once the rice and chicken are cooked, let stand for 10 minutes, covered.

8. Meanwhile, mix the tamari and sesame oil in a serving bowl.

9. Garnish the rice and chicken with cilantro and serve with the sauce.

Ginger Tempeh
Makes 4 servings | 180 calories per serving

Ingredients

• 2 teaspoons cornstarch, potato starch, or kudzu ½ cup vegetable stock

• ½ pound tempeh, cut into ½-inch strips

• 2 tablespoons tamari (gluten-free soy sauce)

• 1 tablespoon shaoshing wine, MMGF or dry sherry

• 1 tablespoon mirin

• 1 tablespoon grapeseed oil

• 2 tablespoons chopped fresh ginger

• 1 small head broccoli, cut into small florets

• 2 tablespoons chopped fresh cilantro or basil, for garnish

• Cooked brown rice, for serving

Direction

1. Preheat the oven to 400°F.

2. Dissolve the cornstarch in the stock and set aside.

3. Place the tempeh on an oiled baking sheet and bake for 20 minutes, or until lightly browned. Set aside.

4. In a bowl, mix the tamari, shaoshing, and mirin and set aside.

5. In a hot wok or frying pan over medium-high heat, add the grapeseed oil.

6. Add the ginger and stir-fry for 30 seconds.

7. Add the broccoli and stir-fry for 3 minutes, or until the vegetable is bright green and slightly soft.

8. Add the tamari mixture and stir-fry for 10 more seconds.

9. Add the dissolved cornstarch and stock and stir-fry for 30 seconds, until it bubbles and thickens.

10. Add the tempeh and stir to coat, cooking until warmed through.

11. Garnish with the cilantro and serve with brown rice.

Tuscan-Style White Pork with Rosemary
Makes 6 servings | 285 calories per serving

Ingredients

• 2 small- to medium-size pork tenderloins

• 1 teaspoon sea salt

• 2–3 tablespoons olive oil

• 1 large bunch fresh rosemary, or 2 handfuls

• 1–1½ quarts low-fat milk

Direction

1. Cut each of the pork tenderloins into three pieces and salt all sides.

2. Heat the oil in a soup pot over medium-high and brown the 6 pork pieces.

3. When the pork pieces are browned, lower the heat to medium and add the rosemary.

4. Cover the rosemary and the meat with milk; this will take about a quart, possibly more.

5. Bring to a slow bubbling boil and cook for 45 minutes.

6. Remove the meat and slice, serving each portion with some of the intact rosemary stems.

Tempeh Marsala

Makes 4 servings | 340 calories per serving

Ingredients

Tempeh

- Bowl one: ½ cup white flour mixed with ¼ teaspoon salt

- Bowl two: ½ cup soymilk mixed with ¼ teaspoon salt

- Bowl three: ½ cup cornmeal mixed with ½ teaspoon salt, ½ teaspoon dried oregano, ½ teaspoon dried rosemary, ½ teaspoon dried thyme, and 2 tablespoons nutritional yeast

• 1 pound tempeh, cut into 8 equal-size cutlets

Marsala

• 2 tablespoons olive oil

• ¼ pound cremini mushrooms, thinly sliced

• 1 cup fresh shelled peas

• 1 teaspoon dried oregano

• 1½ teaspoons sea salt

• ½ cup Marsala wine

• ½ teaspoon black pepper (optional)

• ¼ cup chopped fresh basil

Directions for the Tempeh

1. Preheat the oven to 425°F.

2. Place the 3 bowls in order in a row.

3. Dip a tempeh cutlet once in the flour (bowl one), flip, and dip the other side.

4. Now dip the same cutlet in the soymilk mixture (bowl two), coating both sides, and then dip it in the cornmeal mixture (bowl three), coating both sides.

5. Place the breaded tempeh on a baking sheet lightly coated with oil and repeat with the remaining cutlets.

6. Bake for 30 minutes, or until crisp. (Alternatively, deep-fry until golden brown.)

Directions for the Marsala

1. In a frying pan, heat up the olive oil.

2. Add the mushrooms, peas, oregano, and salt and cook for 5 minutes.

3. Add the Marsala wine, cover, and cook for another 5 minutes, until the alcohol evaporates.

4. Pour over the cutlets.

5. Season with salt and pepper and garnish with basil.

Tofu Cutlets

Makes 4 servings | 160 calories per serving

Ingredients

- 1 pound firm tofu, cut into ½-inch-thick slabs

- ¼ cup cornmeal

- ¼ cup nutritional yeast

- 1 teaspoon sea salt

- 2 tablespoons dried herbs (combination of marjoram, oregano, thyme, basil, sage, rosemary)

- ⅓ cup soymilk or almond milk

- 2 tablespoons olive oil

Direction

1. Preheat the oven to 400°F.

2. Press the tofu by placing the slabs on a towel. Cover with another towel and place a cutting board on the top towel. Place a can or something heavy on the board and let sit for 15 minutes.

3. In a bowl, combine the cornmeal, nutritional yeast, salt, and herbs. Pour the soymilk into a separate bowl.

4. Oil a baking sheet with the olive oil.

5. Dip each piece of tofu in the soymilk and then in the herb-cornmeal mixture, thoroughly coating all sides of each.

6. Place each crusted piece of tofu on the baking sheet, not letting the pieces touch.

7. Bake for 30 minutes, or until nice and crispy.

Basil Chicken
Makes 6 servings | 325 calories per serving

Ingredients

- ¼ cup sesame oil or extra-virgin olive oil

- 10 (⅛-inch-thick) slices peeled fresh ginger

- 2 pounds chicken breast, chopped into bite-size chunks 1 cup rice wine preferably shaoshing, or dry sherry)

- 1 cup tamari (gluten-free soy sauce)

- 2 whole star anise, or 1 tablespoon aniseed

- 1 tablespoon honey

- 1 bunch fresh basil, chopped

- Steamed white rice, for serving

Direction

1. Heat the oil in a pan over medium-high heat, then add the ginger and cook until fragrant, about 1 minute.

2. Add the chicken pieces and brown for 1–2 minutes.

3. Add the rice wine, tamari, star anise, and honey and bring to a boil, then reduce the heat to a simmer and cook for 15 minutes, or until the chicken is cooked through.

4. Stir in the basil and remove from the heat. Serve over rice.

Makes 4 servings | 385 calories per serving

Ingredients

- 1 pound halibut, cut into 4 equal-size pieces

- ½ teaspoon salt

- ½ teaspoon rice wine

- 5 dried shiitake mushrooms

- ¼ cup olive oil

- 4 (⅛-inch-thick) slices peeled fresh ginger

- 10 thin slices prosciutto, chopped

- 10 slices canned bamboo shoots

- 1 cup chicken stock

- 2–4 tablespoons chopped fresh cilantro, for garnish

Direction

1. Marinate the halibut in the salt and rice wine for 10 minutes.

2. Soak the mushrooms in warm water until soft. Rinse the mushrooms and pat dry. Remove the stems and thinly slice the caps.

3. Heat the oil in a pan over medium-high heat, then add the ginger and sauté for 1 minute.

4. Add the mushrooms, prosciutto, and bamboo shoots and sauté for 1 minute.

5. Add the halibut and chicken stock and cover the pan.

6. Poach until the fish is cooked through (poach 10–15 minutes per 1 inch of thickness).

7. Top with cilantro and serve.

Turkey Burger Salad with Black Olives & Avocado
Makes 4 servings | 275 calories per serving

Ingredients

• 1 pound ground turkey (preferably 93% lean/7% fat, as 99% lean can be too dry), formed into 4 patties

• ½ teaspoon sea salt

• 2 heads romaine lettuce, washed and cut or torn into 2- to 3-inch pieces

• 1 medium-size can of small, pitted black olives

• 2 tablespoons extra-virgin olive oil

• 1 teaspoon balsamic vinegar

• 1 avocado, peeled and sliced

Direction

1. Season the turkey patties with the salt and cook on the grill or on the stovetop in a covered frying pan, over medium to medium-high heat for 4–5 minutes per side.

2. After cooking, put the burgers aside until cool enough to break into bite-size pieces.

3. Place the lettuce, olives, oil, and vinegar in a large salad bowl and toss.

4. Finally, add the burger pieces and avocado slices on top.

Gluten-Free Pasta with Shrimp & Zucchini

Makes 6 servings | 460 calories per serving

Ingredients

• 1 pound gluten-free white-rice spaghetti

• 3–4 medium-size zucchinis, halved lengthwise and then sliced into ¼-inch half-moons

• ½ teaspoon sea salt

• 4 tablespoons olive oil

• 1½–2 pounds shrimp (fresh or frozen, uncooked or cooked), peeled and deveined

• ¾ cup chopped fresh basil leaves, stems removed

Direction

1. Get all of the ingredients ready at the start, because the sauce will take about the same time as the pasta to cook. If the shrimp are frozen, defrost them in cold water and then dry them.

2. Put a large pasta pot filled two-thirds with water over high heat.

3. When the water comes to a vigorous, rolling boil, put the pasta in.

4. Start the sauce when the pasta goes into the boiling water.

5. Salt the zucchini. In a large saucepan over high heat, place half of the olive oil and then add the zucchini. Brown the zucchini slices, turning them with a spatula; try not to "boil" them, which is why a big pan and high heat is best.

6. When the zucchini are almost done, add the shrimp. If they are raw, add more of the olive oil, if needed, then add the basil. Cook until heated through.

7. When the pasta is done, drain and serve in individual bowls.

8. Top with the shrimp and zucchini.

Makes 2–4 servings | 210 calories per serving

Ingredients

- 1 pound Arctic char, skin on

- 1–2 teaspoons olive oil

- 1 teaspoon sea salt

- 1 cup chicken or vegetable stock

- 2 teaspoons minced fresh dill, stems removed

Direction

1. Cut the fish in half so that it will fit neatly in your pan, or you may cut it into individual servings.

2. Cover both sides of the fish lightly with the olive oil and then the salt.

3. Heat a shallow pan over medium-high heat, and then add the fish skin-side up.

4. Sauté for 2–3 minutes, until there is some sizzle.

5. Add the chicken stock and half of the dill.

6. When the stock is boiling lightly and steaming, cover the pan with a lid or foil. (If the steaming around the edges of the pan is excessive, lower the heat slightly.)

7. Cook for 12–18 minutes, until the fish skin peels off very easily; that's how you know it is done.

8. Plate and garnish with the rest of the fresh dill.

Watermelon Sorbet

Makes 4 servings | 15 calories per serving

Ingredients

- 4 cups watermelon purée

- 1 tablespoon lemon zest

Direction

1. Combine the watermelon purée and lemon zest and freeze in an ice cream maker according to the manufacturer's instructions.

Ginger-Carrot Ice Pop

Makes 2 servings | 160 calories per serving

Ingredients

- 2 tablespoons agave

- 2 cups fresh carrot juice

• 2 teaspoons fresh ginger juice

Direction

1. Mix all of the ingredients together and pour into an ice pop mold. Insert sticks and freeze until set.

Cucumber Cooler

Makes 4 servings | 20 calories per serving

Ingredients

• 2 cucumbers (preferably Japanese or Persian), peeled

• 4 quarts water

Direction

1. Purée the cucumbers in a blender with a little of the water until smooth.

2. Combine the purée with the rest of the water.

3. Pour over ice and serve.

Cucumber Sorbet

Makes 4 servings | 50 calories per serving

Ingredients

- 2 pounds cucumbers (preferably Japanese or Persian), peeled

- 1 cup water

- 1 teaspoon lemon zest

- 2 tablespoons maple syrup (optional; this works without any sweetener)

Direction

1. Place all of the ingredients in a blender and purée until smooth.

2. Transfer purée to an ice cream maker and churn until frozen according to manufacturer's instructions.

Kick-Ass Carrot Cookies

Makes 3 dozen cookies | 65 calories per cookie

Ingredients

- 1 cup rolled oats

- 1 cup white flour

- 1 teaspoon ground cinnamon

- 1 teaspoon baking powder

- ½ teaspoon baking soda

- ¼ teaspoon salt

- ½ cup maple syrup

- ½ cup grapeseed oil

- 1 cup grated carrot

- ½ cup dried cherries

Direction

1. Preheat the oven to 375°F.

2. In one bowl, combine the oats, flour, cinnamon, baking powder, baking soda, and salt.

3. In a separate bowl, whisk together the syrup and oil.

4. Add the carrots and dried cherries to the wet mixture and mix well.

5. Pour the wet mixture over the dry mixture and gently combine. Do NOT overmix, or the cookies will be rubbery.

6. Drop 1-teaspoon portions of the mixture on a grapeseed-oiled baking sheet, 2 inches apart. (These cookies only bake well if they are small.)

7. Bake for 10 minutes. Be careful not to overcook, as they burn easily.

Makes 2 servings | 75 calories per serving

Ingredients

• 8 (½-inch by ½-inch by 2–3-inch-long) rectangular solids (like square logs), cut from the heart of half a watermelon, avoiding seeds

• 4 thin slices prosciutto

• 2 teaspoons crumbled feta cheese

Direction

1. Place a medium-size frying pan over high heat.

2. When the pan is extremely hot, spray it with nonstick cooking spray and add four of the watermelon logs.

3. Rotate the logs to scan each of the four sides. If the pan is hot enough, it takes around 30 seconds per side. (You only want them to hear a little bit; no more.)

4. Remove from the heat and sit outside when the first four watermelons have a thin layer of black on both sides.

5. Repeat Step 5 with the remaining four watermelon logs.

6. To plate, neatly arrange two pieces of prosciutto on each 8-inch plate, followed by four watermelon logs (two on top of two) for each dish.

7. Garnish each watermelon tower with a teaspoon of feta.

Poached Pears with Tea & Vanilla

Makes 4 servings | 163 calories per serving

Ingredients

- 1 quart water

- 2 vanilla beans, split in half

- 3 cardamom pods

- 1 cinnamon stick

- 2 cloves

- ½ cup maple syrup

- 2 tablespoons jasmine tea leaves, or 4 jasmine tea bags (oolong can be substituted)

- 2 large pears, halved and cored

Direction

1. Bring the water to a boil.

2. Add the vanilla, cardamom, cinnamon, cloves, syrup, and tea.

3. Cover, remove from the heat, and let sit for 10 minutes. Remove the tea (if you have not used tea bags, strain to remove the loose tea leaves).

4. Bring back to a simmer.

5. Add the pears, cover, and cook over low heat for 20 minutes.

Banana Pistachio Ice Cream

Makes 8 servings | 150 calories per serving

Ingredients

- ½ cup raw pistachios

- 2 cups water

- ½ cup maple syrup

- 4 ripe bananas

- ½ teaspoon ground cinnamon

Direction

1. Place all of the ingredients in a blender and purée until totally smooth.

2. Transfer the purée to an ice cream maker and churn until frozen according to the manufacturer's instructions.

Caramelized Bananas

Makes 4 servings | 110 calories per serving

Ingredients

- ¼ cup palm sugar

- ¼ cup water

- 2 bananas, halved lengthwise

Direction

1. In a small frying pan over medium-low heat, combine the sugar and water, stirring until the sugar dissolves.

2. Add the bananas, cook for 5 minutes, and then turn over and cook another 5 minutes.

Natural Fruit Mold

Makes 4 servings | 70 calories per serving

Ingredients

- 2 cups water

- 1 cup fresh blueberry juice

- 2 teaspoons kanten (agar) powder

- Fresh seasonal fruit, sliced

- Seasonal berries

Direction

1. In a saucepan, heat up the water and juice, then add the kanten powder and stir constantly with a whisk to dissolve.

2. Bring the mixture to a boil, lower the heat, and cook, stirring constantly, for 3 minutes.

3. Pour the kanten mixture into a 9 x 13-inch glass baking dish.

4. Decorate with fresh fruit slices and berries.

5. Let set for 2 hours, then chill before serving.

Shaved Fruit Ice

Makes 4 servings | 120 calories per serving

Ingredients

- 4 cups crushed ice

- 4 tablespoons honey

- 4 tablespoons vanilla almond milk

- 2 cups diced seasonal fruits

Direction

1. Divide the crushed ice equally into four serving cups.

2. Drizzle 1 tablespoon honey and 1 tablespoon almond milk over each ice cup.

3. Top each with ½ cup diced fruits.

KITCHEN STAPLES

Garlic-Oil Dressing

Ingredients

- 2 tablespoons garlic-infused olive oil

- 1 teaspoon rice vinegar

- ½ teaspoon sea salt

Direction

1. Whisk all of the ingredients together in a bowl. Store covered in the refrigerator for up to 2 weeks.

Sesame Dressing

Ingredients

- ¼ cup toasted sesame seeds

- 1 tablespoon seaweed-mushroom stock

- 1 ½ tablespoons tamari (gluten-free soy sauce)

- 1 teaspoon sake

- 1 tablespoon mirin

Direction

1. Whisk all of the ingredients together in a bowl. Store covered in the refrigerator for up to 2 weeks.

Chinese Spice Blend

Ingredients

- 1 teaspoon ground cinnamon

- ½ teaspoon ground cloves

- 1 teaspoon fennel seeds, toasted and ground

- 1 teaspoon ground aniseed

- ½ teaspoon ground ginger

Direction

1. Mix all of the ingredients together in an airtight container and store for up to 1 month.

Ingredients

• Handful of garlic cloves, peeled

• Olive oil

Direction

1. Place several garlic cloves in olive oil (they should be covered) and let sit for a few days at room temperature.

2. Remove the cloves and discard.

3. Store the oil in the refrigerator and use within 2 weeks.

Ingredients

• 5 pounds cabbage, shredded

• 3 tablespoons sea salt

Direction

1. Place the cabbage in a bowl and sprinkle with the salt.

2. Massage the salt into the cabbage for a few minutes, making sure that the cabbage is completely covered with the salt.

3. Pack the salted cabbage tightly into a crock.

4. Place a weight on the cabbage to keep it submerged in the liquid that it will expel as it ferments.

5. Cover loosely and let sit in a clean area for 1 month.

6. Skim off the top layer and enjoy the kraut.

Vegetable Stock

Ingredients

- 3 dried shiitake mushrooms

- 1 carrot, peeled and coarsely chopped

- 1 stalk celery, coarsely chopped

- 1 potato, peeled and coarsely chopped

- ¼ cup parsley stems

- 2–3 (6-inch) square pieces kombu (a type of Japanese seaweed; optional)

- 1 teaspoon sea salt

- 2 quarts water

Direction

1. In a small stockpot, add the mushrooms, carrot, celery, potato, parsley stems, kombu, salt, and water.

2. Bring to a boil, cover, lower the heat, and let simmer for 30 minutes.

3. Simmer longer for a deeper flavor.

Chicken Stock

Ingredients

- 5 quarts cold water

- 4 ½–5-pound chicken, cut into 8 pieces, excess skin and fat removed

- 1 tablespoon salt

- 1-pound yam, peeled, halved crosswise

- ¾ pound carrots, peeled, thickly sliced

- ½ pound parsnips, peeled, thickly sliced

- 4 large stalks celery, cut into 2-inch pieces

- 12 large fresh dill sprigs

- 12 large fresh parsley sprigs

- Lemon zest of 1 lemon

Direction

1. Bring the water to a boil in a stockpot.

2. Add the chicken and return to a boil, skimming any impurities, for 15 minutes. Add the yam, carrots, parsnips, and celery. Reduce the heat to medium-low and gently simmer for 1 ½ hours.

3. Add the dill, parsley, and lemon zest and simmer for 3 minutes.

4. Remove from the heat and let stand for an hour, then strain. Store stock in the refrigerator for up to 2 days or freeze for up to 1 month.

Seaweed-Mushroom Stock (kombu dashi)

1. A very easy and flavorful stock that can be used in almost all savory dishes requiring stock. This is the base stock for my other stocks. By adding more ingredients (vegetables, vegetable parts, spices, herbs), we can produce very different-flavored stocks.

2. Seaweed-mushroom stock uses two inexpensive Japanese ingredients, both easy to find at Japanese or Asian markets and at many grocery stores. These days, we can easily find any ingredient online.

Ingredients

• 3 dried shiitake mushrooms

- 2–3 6-inch square pieces kombu (a type of Japanese seaweed)

- 1 teaspoon sea salt

- 2 quarts water

Direction

1. In a small stockpot, add the mushrooms, kombu, and water.

2. Bring to a boil, cover, lower the heat, and let simmer for 30 minutes.

3. Simmer longer for a deeper flavor.

4. Once you have seaweed-mushroom stock, you can make Miso Soup (page 109) in a couple of minutes.

Balsamic Vinegar & Oil Dressing

Ingredients

- 2 tablespoons balsamic vinegar

- 2 tablespoons olive oil

- ¼ teaspoon dried thyme

- ¼ teaspoon dried marjoram or oregano

- ½ teaspoon mustard powder

- ¼ teaspoon sea salt

Direction

1. Whisk all of the ingredients together in a bowl. Store covered in the refrigerator for up to 2 weeks.

CONCLUSION

The Silent Reflux Diet is a comprehensive approach to managing the symptoms of laryngopharyngeal reflux (LPR) and preventing further complications.

While it may require significant lifestyle changes and dietary modifications, the benefits of adhering to this diet can be far-reaching and life-changing for those suffering from the debilitating effects of silent reflux.

One of the primary advantages of the Silent Reflux Diet is its potential to alleviate symptoms without the need for long-term medication or invasive procedures.

By carefully selecting and avoiding specific foods and beverages, individuals can effectively reduce the frequency and severity of reflux episodes, thereby mitigating the damage to the throat, larynx, and vocal cords.

However, it's important to recognize that the Silent Reflux Diet is not a quick fix or a one-size-fits-all solution.

Successful implementation of this dietary approach requires patience, diligence, and a willingness to make sustainable lifestyle changes. Keeping a detailed food diary and closely monitoring symptom patterns can be invaluable in identifying personal trigger foods and making appropriate adjustments to the diet.

While the initial transition to the Silent Reflux Diet may be challenging, particularly for those accustomed to consuming acidic, spicy, or fried foods, the long-term benefits can be profound. By reducing the exposure of the delicate throat tissues to harmful stomach acids and irritants, individuals may experience a significant improvement in their overall quality of life.

The Silent Reflux Diet not only addresses the physical symptoms of LPR but can also have a positive impact on mental well-being. Chronic coughing, hoarseness, and the sensation of a lump in the throat can be emotionally taxing, leading to anxiety, frustration, and social withdrawal. By effectively managing these symptoms, individuals may regain confidence in their ability to communicate clearly and participate in social interactions without discomfort or embarrassment.

Moreover, the Silent Reflux Diet emphasizes the consumption of nutrient-dense, whole foods that can contribute to overall health and well-being. The emphasis on lean proteins, complex carbohydrates, and non-acidic fruits and vegetables can provide a balanced and nourishing dietary foundation, potentially reducing the risk of other chronic conditions associated with poor dietary habits.

It's important to note that while the Silent Reflux Diet can be an effective management strategy, it may not be suitable for everyone. Individuals with specific dietary restrictions, such as food allergies or intolerances, may require additional modifications or guidance from a healthcare professional or registered dietitian. Additionally, those with severe or persistent symptoms may require additional treatment options, such as medication or surgical intervention, in conjunction with dietary changes.

The success of the Silent Reflux Diet ultimately relies on a collaborative approach between the individual, healthcare providers, and support systems. Seeking guidance from a knowledgeable healthcare team, including a gastroenterologist, speech-language pathologist, and registered dietitian, can ensure that the diet is tailored to individual needs and that any potential nutrient deficiencies or imbalances are addressed.

Furthermore, enlisting the support of family and friends can be instrumental in maintaining adherence to the diet. Having a strong support system can provide encouragement, accountability, and a shared understanding of the challenges and benefits associated with the Silent Reflux Diet.

In conclusion, the Silent Reflux Diet is a comprehensive and potentially life-changing approach to managing the symptoms of laryngopharyngeal reflux. While it may require significant lifestyle adjustments and ongoing commitment, the potential benefits of alleviating chronic symptoms, preventing further complications, and improving overall quality of life make it a valuable consideration for those affected by this condition. By working closely with healthcare professionals, staying diligent, and fostering a supportive environment, individuals can successfully navigate the challenges of the Silent Reflux Diet and experience the profound relief it can provide.